12 KEYS TO ENJOYING A HEALTHY LIFE

JOYCE MEYER

INTRODUCTION

Do you have any idea how valuable you are? Maybe you never learned your own importance. Or maybe you did know your value when you were younger, but somewhere along the way you forgot it. If so, join the club.

The degraded value systems in the modern world bombard us with the message that our spirit, soul, and body come last, after money and food and status and stuff. Reforming your value system to *God's* value system puts your entire being (body, mind, will, emotions, and spirit) right at the top of God's list of important and valuable things.

To be effective for the Kingdom, we need to be at the top of our game. We are tri-part beings and have many facets to our nature, each needing proper care.

All your ability to be active and do good in the world requires a healthy mind, body, and soul, and those things rely on a healthy lifestyle and environment. Keeping this big picture in mind can help you stay on your life's path.

I am teaching on this subject because I am dismayed at the number of people I see—at my book signings, in my ministry, and in the general public—who are not taking care of themselves. If it is in our nature to take care of ourselves, then *why don't we*? After some thought, I came up with these reasons:

1. WE DON'T KNOW HOW TO TAKE CARE OF OUR PHYSICAL BODIES.

People are confused about what a wholesome diet is and how they should eat. I'll give you the information you need and some simple guidelines.

2. WE HAVE A SKEWED BODY IMAGE PLANTED IN OUR MINDS BY MEDIA AND ADVERTISING.

On the one hand we are presented with unattainable ideals of beauty, while on the other hand obesity is so prevalent it has nearly become the norm. We need to reset our internal picture of what a healthy person should look like.

3. WE HAVE LOST TOUCH WITH EXERCISE.

For virtually all of human existence, exercise was an integral part of our daily existence. Now we've invented enough conveniences that we often live completely divorced from exercise. However, it turns out a good deal of our well-being is dependent on exercise.

4. WE HAVE LET OURSELVES SLIP INTO UNWORKABLE LIVES.

We have developed lifestyles that encourage us to shortchange nutrition, sleep, and relationships. Life is a gift, and it is meant to be pleasurable and sane.

5. SOME HAVE BECOME PATHOLOGICALLY SELFLESS.

We are to live sacrificially and be involved in doing good works, but we must not ignore our own basic needs in the process. Everything in life must be balanced or something breaks down and quite often, it is us.

6. WE HAVE LOST OUR SUPPORT.

Maintaining a good support network is a terrific way to prevent the formation of bad habits. We need to have the right people around us who will speak up if they see us getting out of balance.

7. WE HAVE FORGOTTEN OUR OWN VALUE.

Reminding you of your place in God's plan is my first and most important task. God has a great future planned for you and you need to be ready for it! You need to look great and feel great, ready to do whatever God asks of you.

MY STORY

First Corinthians 6:19–20 explains that your body is the temple of the Holy Spirit. You may well feel that temple is in shambles and have no idea how to begin the restoration process. I know that feeling.

My poor relationship with my body began with sexual, emotional, and mental abuse throughout my childhood. During those years, I developed a shame-based nature and felt bad about myself all the time.

At the age of eighteen, I married, left home, and moved more than fifteen times in a five-year period. My first marriage was extremely stressful, and we separated numerous times. My husband was a heavy drinker, had affairs with other women, and was a petty thief. I can't begin to describe how unstable my life was back then.

After the birth of my first son, I divorced my husband and had nowhere to go, so I lived with relatives for a while and then moved back in with my parents out of desperation. I'm sure you can see that stress was my normal state. I did not realize that all of this was taking its toll on my body.

Nine months later, I met Dave Meyer. The first years of our marriage were very difficult. He was a committed Christian or I doubt he would have stayed with me. Though my relationship with God then was not what I now call healthy, I worked hard at it—as I did at everything. I wanted to help people and God called me into ministry at age thirty-three.

As a woman trying to start a new ministry, I experienced opposition from friends, family, and my church. More stress! I threw myself into my ministry full-tilt, and I concentrated hard on success. Sleep? Relaxation? Fun? Laughter? To me, this was like wasting time.

By the time I was thirty-six, my body was showing symptoms of exhaustion. I got sick for four months straight. Then I developed various problems related to my hormones and menstrual cycle, culminating in a hysterectomy.

In 1989 I was diagnosed with breast cancer which required immediate surgery. The surgery was successful, but it led to my hormonal system being more messed up than ever, which led to several more years of misery. During this time, my migraine headaches started. They were regular and excruciating.

Despite all of this, I continued my work in the ministry. I traveled, taught God's Word, stood in faith for my own healing, and often wondered how I could go on much longer. I was so tired inside and out that when I woke up in the morning I wished it was time to go to bed. I did my duty, I worked hard, but I did not enjoy *anything*.

For years, while my ministry grew and flourished, I was constantly sick. It was rarely completely debilitating, but it was one small thing after another. I never, ever felt truly well. My body tried to tell me something, but I didn't listen.

I finally came to a point when I was so depleted that if anything stressful happened I would experience shortness of breath and break into a sweat. I even cried easily, and my body and emotions felt completely alien to me. When my blood pressure hit a dangerous peak, I knew it was time to make some changes.

When I finally combined nutritional help with positive lifestyle changes, I started seeing good results. But this didn't happen overnight! It took almost three years before I felt really good. But my health improved gradually all along the way, and just receiving a taste of being better is a powerful motivator.

Don't settle for feeling bad one more day. There is help! Your body has the ability to restore itself if you follow God's guidelines for good health.

I wrote my book, *Look Great, Feel Great* because I can truthfully say that I feel better physically, mentally, emotionally, and spiritually right now than I ever have in my life. I live every day passionately, and what a breathtaking change that is.

These are my best days. I have an energy and contentment I have never known, a fierce faith, and I fully expect to live out my life in health and grace. This is your birthright as well, and I hope you'll join with me as we take up our spiritual hammers and begin your restoration.

AMERICA'S SELF-RESPECT CRISIS

Look around America, and you will see the many signs of a society in the throes of a self-respect crisis. I believe there is a connection between low self-esteem and an unwillingness to make any investment in taking care of ourselves.

People with healthy self-esteem are more likely to take

care of themselves. People who take the time to do the little things to make themselves look and feel good are more likely to hold a positive self-image. They are more likely to make better parents, more loving partners, quality workers, and smarter entrepreneurs.

Look great, feel great. Feel great, look great. It's no coincidence that the two often go together.

The Wisdom of Investing in Your Health

There are two groups I hope to reach with this message: the people who have given up on themselves and the overachievers who believe they can't be bothered by little things like diet and exercise.

Don't refuse to do maintenance and run your body into the ground (the grave) earlier than God intended. Like any other kind of investment, investing in yourself demands some of your resources. In terms of money, it demands very little. The larger investment may be your time.

Looking Nice Is Not a Sin

"Does God really care what I look like? Do I have to be thin?" God cares most that you go forth clothed in righteousness. But righteousness *plus* a nice outfit never hurt anyone. If people see that you respect yourself, they respect you, too.

Like everything else in life, it is a question of balance. Keep the big picture in mind. Ask yourself, "What is the work that God has put me on earth to do?" Then decide what amount of attention you should pay to how you look and feel to get the maximum energy, health, and charisma you need to do that work as successfully as possible.

Remember, in order for you to achieve success in these areas, you have to do more than read . . . you must also act on it!

Be doers of the Word, and not hearers only.
(James 1:22 NKJV)

KEY 1 LET GOD DO THE HEAVY LIFTING

We've all had the experience. Whether the goal in question is a weight loss diet, an exercise routine, a change in how we treat other people, or any other self-improvement mission, failure makes us turn on ourselves. Soon we are wallowing in a pit of self-pity and disgust.

The Truth About Willpower

We criticize ourselves for a lack of willpower, believing that if we had enough of it we could fight off every temptation that came our way. Here's a little secret about willpower. It is your best friend when things go well, but it's the first friend to check out when you get weary.

Willpower and discipline are important and vitally necessary to a successful life, but willpower alone won't be enough. Determination gets you started and keeps you going for awhile, but it is never enough to bring you across the finish line.

Now, what happens if, instead of turning first to willpower in your time of need, you turn to God instead? God releases His power into your willpower and energizes it to bring you across the finish line. Willpower does not get the credit for our success, God does. Jesus said in John 15:5, "Apart from Me you can do nothing."

We must learn to let God do the heavy lifting. Let Him supply the ability to energize our choices. We can choose to exercise or stop overeating, but our choice alone is not enough for complete victory.

Breaking Your Bonds

God has an awesome plan for you, but it requires you to learn the power you have as His child and begin exercising it. You can break out of old behavior patterns and live in freedom, but too often we instead prefer the ease of familiar bonds. A prisoner who feels safe in his cell may stay in it, even when we fling open the door to his freedom.

When you are struggling for the umpteenth time to lose weight, that first step seems like the heaviest one in the world. A short-term diet may appear easier, and you may experience some temporary success, but what we truly desire is permanent freedom. If you turn things over to God, the Source of Divine Strength, you will finally find the power you need to break free.

Draw on the limitless power of the Holy Spirit, rather than your own very limited power. He will always lead you to victory and freedom.

SCIENCE CATCHES ON

You don't have to take my word about God's ability to help you succeed. Even science is finally starting to come around to the fact that faith works.

According to recent studies, churchgoers are more successful at overcoming alcoholism and smoking, they are more likely to get exercise, and they are less likely to be depressed. Not surprisingly, they also have a longer life expectancy than non-churchgoers.

FIVE WAYS TO TRUST GOD WITH YOUR BURDENS

1. ASK

You need to take the time to quiet your mind and open it to God. Ask Him to be your partner in your personal restoration. You will be amazed at what a huge difference it makes to directly invite God into your life to help solve problems.

2. ATTEND CHURCH

Most of us find that the weekly boost of prayer, education, community, and sacred space we get at church gives us a far stronger bond. If you are struggling for ways to make contact with God, and you haven't tried church yet, what are you waiting for?

3. ATTEND A SUPPORT GROUP

If you work best when you can share your struggle with others who are going through the same thing, then seek out a support group. They can help you admit you are powerless and encourage you to turn your restoration over to God.

4. BEGIN EACH DAY WITH AN AFFIRMATION

First thing when you wake up in the morning, take a moment to renew your commitment to God and refresh your spirit with His strength. Write an affirmation that is based on Bible promises and addresses your specific needs . . . then daily speak it out with confidence.

5. PRAY IN MOMENTS OF DOUBT

No matter who you are, you will find moments when your determination weakens. When you get that feeling, don't quit, but don't blindly bull forward in your own strength, either. Step back, take a moment, and ask God to carry you through.

TAKING ACTION

Choose at least one action you can take to begin letting God do the heavy lifting.

NOTES:

KEY 2   LEARNING TO LOVE YOUR BODY

What if everywhere you went, you ran into someone you didn't like? Wouldn't that be terrible? "Oh no," you'd think, "her again?" That sounds pretty awful, but that's exactly your situation if you don't like yourself, because you are everywhere you go.

I'm amazed at how few people are truly at peace with themselves. Instead, they have declared war on themselves, and the cause, frequently, is the body. Here are some of the factors that cause us to hate our bodies.

Abuse in Childhood

Small children instinctively feel comfortable with how they look. But mistreatment can undermine that natural understanding of the body so that it becomes the source of emotional pain.

I know this firsthand.

Abuse doesn't have to be sexual or physical to cause these problems. Authority figures or even peers are perfectly capable of driving home the message that we are bad or useless and that our bodies are ugly and evil. Until you confront your feelings, you will be in a constant state of warfare with yourself, experiencing the stress, trauma, and exhaustion that war always causes.

Misunderstanding the Bible's Teachings

The Bible tells us to resist the flesh and embrace the spirit, but that doesn't mean hate the flesh! Too many people believe they would be fine if not for that awful flesh tempting and confusing them. They blame the body for interfering with their spiritual development and wish they could just get rid of it. They forget that the body is the temple for the Holy Spirit. Use your body to bring glory to God.

Media Messages

Do you resemble the models you see in magazines and on billboards? Neither do I! Don't spend your life competing with an illusion! Don't live in the agony of unrealistic expectations! I'm at peace with my body. I strongly believe in taking what we have to work with and doing the most we can with it. I try to look my best, but I don't allow myself to be pressured by unrealistic expectations.

The Beauty Industry

It's the beauty industry's job to make you feel that you need their products. The truth is, you are already beautiful in God's eyes, and if you follow His principles, you will look better on the outside. I look better than I did twenty years ago because I worry less and am happier; therefore, I look more refreshed.

Take better care of yourself beginning today. If you know God and understand your own value, you will not be desperate for the newest beauty cream or program.

Age and Sickness

You can be comfortable with your looks and immune to the spells of the beauty industry, and still fall out of love with your body as you age. Exercise and staying active will help, but you also need to develop a realistic picture of what you should look and feel like at that stage of life. Determine to be the best "you" that you can, and stop trying to be what the world says you should be.

FIVE WAYS TO NURTURE SELF-LOVE

1. DON'T CHASE YOUR YOUTH

People who long for their youth are never content, because every day that youth gets a little farther away. It's better to enjoy who you are now and try to live and look appropriate for someone your age. And remember, no matter how old you are, there is someone older who would love to be as young as you. Cheer up and make the best of things!

2. LEARN TO RECEIVE GOD'S LOVE

The greatest gift that can be given is offered to each of us every day, yet few have the faith and self-esteem to accept it. Think of a wide receiver catching a football pass. He wants that ball and goes after it. That's how to receive God's love. Be passionate about it. Receiving God's love is an important step because we can't love others without it.

3. FOCUS ON THE JOURNEY, NOT THE DESTINATION

I spent many miserable years never enjoying where I was because I was too focused on where I wanted to be. I finally learned that life is about the journey, not the destination, and then the ride became much more fun. Be proud of today's successes. Don't look at how far you have to go but rather how far you've come.

4. LEARN THE FACTS

I believe we need to be more health-conscious than weight-conscious. I am not suggesting that we should be overweight and just not care. But the most important thing is to be healthy and fit. I firmly believe that if we concentrate on good health we will ultimately weigh what is right for us as individuals.

5. VIEW YOUR BODY AS A FRIEND

If you had a friend who was sick or in need, you would do everything you could to help them. That is the attitude you should have toward your body. Do everything you can to help it; don't despise or fight it.

TAKING ACTION

Choose at least one action you can take to nurture self-love.

ACTION:

KEY 3 MASTERING METABOLISM

The Secret to Stable Weight

Did you know that you own a masterpiece? The truth is, you were born with one. Your body is God's masterwork designed to adapt to and survive a variety of situations.

One of the ways your body adapts is through *metabolism*, the process by which your body breaks down or *metabolizes* your food and converts it into energy. We literally burn the food to power ourselves, just as your car burns gasoline for power. We can burn our food or "fuel" at different rates, from extremely fast, hurtling down the highway in overdrive, to very slow, just barely inching forward in first gear.

But that's the danger. If you aren't using much energy but are still "filling up your tank" with as much food as usual, you are in trouble. If you kept putting more gas in your car than you used, the extra would spill out the top of the tank. But remember, our bodies are way more sophisticated than a car. It has an incredible flexible system for storing as much fuel as it can get. Millions of special, flexible cells throughout your body swell up with the extra fuel, saving it for later. Great system, right? Well, yes, but you might not think it's so great when I tell you the name of these cells: fat cells. These cells are how the body efficiently stores energy for later.

The body also tries to be careful about the rate at which it uses these resources. If it doesn't get much food (or water), it assumes that hard times are here and slows down your metabolism. Great if you're on a desert island, but terrible if you are on a diet.

Why Diets Backfire

You can see why diets wreck metabolism. The only way to lose weight is to burn more calories per day than we consume, but as

I just explained, your body's natural instinct is not to keep reviving your metabolism once your food intake goes way down. Not long after you start dieting, it's going to lower your metabolism to match the new amount of food coming in.

It's the classic dieting dilemma: You have great success the first few weeks, but then, even though you are sticking (with difficulty) to the diet and eating like a bird, suddenly the weight loss stops. Soon you start sneaking forbidden food, and the weight comes back with a vengeance. You even seem to have more fat than before!

When your metabolism is slow and you aren't doing much, you tend to lose muscle. If you work a muscle it gets bigger; the less you use it the more it shrinks. Your shape is some combination of muscle and fat. Muscle looks great, stays firm, and flexes when you move. Fat has all the shape of a water balloon. But more importantly, muscle burns calories all the time, just keeping itself ready for action. The more muscle you have, the more calories you burn, *even when sleeping.*

Dieting is not the way to get to, or maintain, a healthy weight. The key is to eat a balanced diet and engage in activities that keep your metabolism purring.

FIVE WAYS TO BOOST METABOLISM

1. EXERCISE

Just as your body interprets dieting as a food shortage and lowers your metabolism to help out, it also assumes that if you move fast every day, you have a good reason; it must be key to your survival. So it raises metabolism, builds muscle, and provides the enzymes that burn calories more easily.

2. EAT BREAKFAST (AND LUNCH AND DINNER)

You've heard that breakfast is the most important meal of the day. It's true! Your metabolism naturally slows down overnight, so breakfast is your body's signal to kick-start itself. Make sure you get some lean protein at breakfast along with some fruit or vegetables for vitamins and fiber. Don't skip lunch or dinner either, but try changing your usual pattern and make dinner the lightest meal of the day.

3. DRINK WATER

Without water you have less energy, because water moves nutrients from your food to your muscles and brain—via blood, which is mostly water. Water gets nutrients to our cells, cools us off, flushes waste, and circulates immune cells through the body. Without water, all these systems suffer. In addition, according to one German study, metabolism rose by 30 percent after drinking two glasses of water and stayed that way for an hour!

4. SLEEP WELL

During sleep, your body is hard at work doing vital maintenance. Skip this stage and you drag through the day with less energy and lowered metabolism. People tend to eat more when sleep-deprived because they feel colder and less energetic and mistake these feelings for hunger.

5. FIDGET

That's right. It's not just the planned exercise that makes the difference, but the hundreds of tiny movements we make, or don't make, throughout the day. Try taking the little conveniences out of your life—take the stairs, don't use the drive-thru, park at the back of the lot.

TAKING ACTION

Choose at least one action you can take to boost your metabolism.

ACTION:

KEY 4 EXERCISE

Whenever the word "exercise" is mentioned, everybody groans. I'll tell you a secret: I groan too!

Very few of us have jobs that involve exercise, and most of our leisure activities are spent with our feet up, too. This is a new development, and a deadly one.

Yes, regular exercise will help you lose weight and look your best, but there are many other benefits. Other than not smoking, nothing can improve your health more. It is truly a magic bullet!

Keeping the Fires Burning

The fuel that powers your body is sugar. A particular kind of sugar called glucose is what your muscles and brain use to keep going. But muscles can't store much glucose; only enough for a few quick actions. After that, they need to reload. The signal goes out to your body for more fuel. That fuel is stored in your body in the form of fat.

The process of breaking down fat requires oxygen. That makes it easy to tell when your muscles have used up their own glucose and are getting more fuel from fat: you start to breathe harder, because you need the oxygen. Any time you feel yourself breathing hard during a workout, pat yourself on the back; it means you are literally burning fat. However, you don't want to exercise so hard that you are *gasping* for breath, because then your body can't keep up with your oxygen demands. And when this happens, it leaves behind a nasty waste product called lactic acid.

The Heart of the Matter

Your energy level depends on getting oxygen and fuel to your muscles, and both of those things are accomplished through the bloodstream. Blood is your transportation network, and your heart drives that network.

When you exercise, the demand for fuel and air increases. Your heart pumps faster and faster to deliver the fuel and oxygen through the bloodstream. Your heart is a muscle like all the others. As it gets used, it gets bigger and stronger and delivers the needed fuel and oxygen with less stress and more efficiency.

At the same time, when you exercise, a thin layer of muscle in your arteries dilates so that more blood can get through. Exercise keeps those arterial muscles strong and flexible so they can dilate wide when needed, and they are less likely to develop dangerous cholesterol buildups and blockages. Now you understand why exercise is so important and can cut your risk of heart attack and stroke in half!

The Diabetes Epidemic

Diabetes is a sugar disease caused by high levels of glucose in the blood—the result of a diet high in fat, sugars, and starches, along with a sedentary lifestyle. Sugary, sticky blood can damage artery walls and forms the clots that cause cardiovascular disease.

Insulin is a hormone that signals muscle cells to open up and absorb more glucose. When the muscles are stuffed, they begin to resist absorption of glucose. This is called "insulin resistance." Then your body turns the glucose to fat and crams it into fat cells. But they start to resist after a while, too. Assuming more and more sugars and starches are coming in by way of mouth, glucose levels in the blood keep rising, and the pancreas pumps out insulin faster and faster. But there's nowhere for the glucose to go, and eventually the pancreas breaks down. Then there is NO way of getting any glucose into muscle cells, and you have a full-blown case of diabetes.

Exercise helps your muscles burn off their glucose supply so they can accept a refill and it reduces insulin resistance.

Cancer and the Immune System

Exercise can reduce your risk of some cancers by stimulating your immune defense, centered in the lymphatic system. The lymph system circulates white blood cells through the body where they find and eliminate threats, like cancer cells. The faster those white blood cells circulate, the more cancer cells they can stop.

Stress and Depression

Stress is simply anything that requires us to react. Our body responds by producing performance-enhancing hormones like adrenaline and cortisol. They help us think faster, react quicker, and have extra strength. This is great if we have some outlet for reacting, like running, delivering a performance on stage, or in some other way being active. However, without a physical outlet, they remain bottled up inside. Exercise burns up those extra hormones and gets our bodies back to a relaxed state. It also triggers the release of endorphins, the chemicals that are responsible for good moods. Our self-esteem is also boosted when we exercise and that too can reduce depression.

Osteoporosis

Bones use calcium as their building blocks, and the more the muscles attached to the bone get used, the stronger your body makes those bones by reinforcing them with extra calcium. But if your bones aren't frequently "tested" by the force of muscle upon them, your body assumes they aren't vital, and it doesn't reinforce them. Regular exercise can preserve your bone strength.

FIVE WAYS TO GET STARTED

1. A DAILY WALK

Something as simple as 30 minutes of walking (about two miles) at a moderate pace will increase your longevity.

2. INDOOR EXERCISE

Don't let the weather keep you from exercising.
Find a fun exercise video.

3. STRENGTH TRAINING

Aerobic exercise improves cardiovascular function, but help for osteoporosis requires strength training such as weight lifting.

4. RUNNING OR BIKING

If you are bored with walking, try running or biking. Biking can be easier on your joints. It can also be a way to accomplish neighborhood errands.

5. SWIMMING

Even if walking isn't possible for you, try swimming. Indoor pools make it a year-round option.

TAKING ACTION

Choose at least one action you can take to get more exercise in your life.

ACTION:

KEY 5 BALANCED EATING

God's very simple dining instructions to Adam and Eve were: "You may freely eat of every tree in the garden" (Genesis 2:16).

Bad diet information has clouded the very simple truths of healthy eating: eat the foods that come from God in as close a state as possible to how God made them, and you can't go wrong.

You are free to eat! Diets fail because they are all about restrictions, rules, and directives. The spirit longs for freedom. Begin a joyful, guilt-free routine of freely eating the good foods God has put on earth for you.

The Low-Fat Catastrophe

Because ounce for ounce, fat has twice as many calories as protein or carbohydrates, researchers told us to cut the fat and replace it with other foods. Most often, those "other foods" were carbohydrates like potatoes, bread, sweets, or pasta. They have fewer calories, but we weren't as satisfied so we ate more. As a result, our blood sugar levels soared as did our rate of diabetes.

Letting the Body Do Its Job

Until a few hundred years ago, there were very few convenient forms of carbohydrates to eat. There was fruit in season, but most other carbohydrates came from vegetables and whole grains, foods that require the digestive system to strip away the fibrous material and more slowly deliver glucose to the bloodstream—and that means blood sugar levels stay nice and steady. Then somebody came along and invented machines that stripped off the chewy outer part of the grain, leaving the soft inner part. White flour is an example. There is no doubt that we love foods made with white flour, but these are the types of foods that cause massive insulin response which leads to overeating, obesity, and diabetes. Eat your food in as natural a state as possible. Make your body do the work it was made for.

Does Fat Make Me Fat?

Fat has compounds in it called leptins that make the body feel full and signal us to stop eating. Yes, fat is a more concentrated form of calories, but we tend to eat it in small amounts. Just like high-fiber whole grains, a little keeps our bodies working longer.

Does Fat Make Me Sick?

Our bodies manufacture cholesterol from the fat in the food we eat. If it is the "bad" LDL cholesterol, it can clog arteries and cause heart attacks and strokes. Switching from saturated to unsaturated fat can lower bad cholesterol and make a huge difference.

Other Benefits of Fat and Natural Fats

We haven't even mentioned the most important benefit of fat, which is that it tastes great! Food that doesn't have flavor isn't satisfying and can cause us to turn to less healthy foods that get us the contentment we are craving.

Rather than less fat, your goal should be to cut saturated fat from your diet and replace it with unsaturated fat in a form that is as close as possible to how God provided it.

Protein

To keep yourself operating at peak efficiency and rebuild tissue as it breaks down, you need a steady supply of protein. Look for sources other than red meat.

Nature's Pharmacy

Many of the things we eat not only supply us with energy, they also have healing qualities. Different types of antioxidants are found in all fruits and vegetables, and they protect different parts of the body from the damage done by free radicals and other toxins in the environment. They bind with toxins, neutralize them, and remove them.

Balance

Look for that balance on your plate. Allow yourself some carbohydrates for energy—preferably whole-grain ones like brown rice, whole wheat, corn kernels, or beans—but make sure they are balanced by plenty of protein and healthy fat.

FIVE WAYS TO PRACTICE BALANCED EATING

1. MAKE FOOD SACRED

Learn to do everything, including eating, for God's glory. Look at your dinner plate and ask if what you are about to eat is mostly what God created for you. Make good choices! Each time you choose good, healthy foods, you are choosing life, which is God's gift to you.

2. AVOID REFINED CARBOHYDRATES

Much of America's obesity is caused by the amount of refined carbohydrates we eat. Let's make it simple: always choose the side salad or vegetable instead of the fries.

3. BE FIERCE ABOUT FRUITS & VEGETABLES
Choose your restaurants by their vegetables. Don't let them take the cheap way by filling you up on bread and chips.

4. SWITCH TO UNSATURATED FATS
Eat less red meat, dairy, and processed foods, and eat more fish, olive oil, nuts, and avocados.

5. BALANCE YOUR PLATE
You can most likely eat all of the foods you love, but you may just need to change the ratio.

TAKING ACTION

Choose at least one action you can take to eat more healthy foods.

ACTION:

KEY 6 WATER YOUR LIFE

You are two-thirds water, just as the earth is two-thirds water and one-third dry land. Water is fundamental to our existence. Without water, energy can't get from your food to your muscles and brain, waste can't get cleansed, kidneys can't function, and the immune system can't circulate.

Even low-grade dehydration has important consequences: fatigue, grumpiness and weak concentration. Don't rely on thirst to tell you when you need more water. We can get used to all kinds of feelings and low-level dehydration can be one of them.

Water and Weight Loss

Water can help you with your weight-loss goals. This is partly because of water's ability to increase metabolism, as I mentioned earlier. Water also can fill your stomach—temporarily, and help you slow down your eating.

Since mild dehydration registers as fatigue and poor concentration rather than thirst, many people mistake the feeling for hunger. They end up snacking throughout the day, when all they really need is a tall glass of water to revive them.

But the biggest reason water is a weight-loss godsend is because when you are drinking water, you are not drinking the other stuff—sodas, shakes, high-calorie coffee drinks, and so on.

If you have spent most of your life consuming sugary drinks, it will take time for your taste buds to adjust to the taste of water. But adjust they will! How much water do you need? One formula is to take your weight, divide by two, and consume that many ounces of liquid a day.

What About Caffeine?

I love my coffee, but because at one time my body was so stressed, I cut out caffeine entirely for a period of time.

Caffeine makes all the classic changes happen in your body that occur in response to any physical or mental stress: the heartbeat quickens, breathing increases, senses sharpen, and your brain picks up speed. This feels good, as do lots of other gentle stressors, like exercise, amusement park rides, and even falling in love! It's only when stress is out of control that it becomes a problem and causes insomnia, disease, and premature aging.

That's what happened to me. I was running myself ragged and coffee only added fuel to the fire. So I cut it out. But once I made lifestyle changes to reduce my stress to normal levels, I discovered to my great joy that I could drink a little coffee each day with no repercussions.

Caffeine has some positive affects. It can reduce your chances of developing kidney stones, gallstones, and depression. And according to a 2005 study, it is America's biggest source of antioxidants. But caffeine is addictive; stopping cold turkey can give you a nasty headache.

Other Drinks

Anything you guzzle can count toward your liquid intake goals, but some may come with a nasty and unnecessary caloric wallop. Sodas, sweetened teas, and "energy drinks" are just sugar water in disguise. Fruit juices have vitamins but are high in calories. Skim milk is an excellent beverage; whole milk, however, is very high in saturated fat.

Fortunately, every convenience store has good bottled water for sale, and sparkling water for those who want to liven things up a bit. There are diet drinks, but health concerns have been raised about the artificial sweeteners. Personally, I stick to drinks with a long safety record: water, sparkling water, coffee, herbal tea, and an occasional fruit juice.

FIVE WAYS TO STAY HYDRATED

1. MAKE IT TASTE GOOD

Do what you have to do to make your drinking something to

look forward to. Put a filter on your tap, squeeze a wedge of lemon into your glass, or make iced herbal tea.

2. CARRY WATER EVERYWHERE
I carry water to business meetings, in the car—you name it.

3. HAVE YOUR WATER CALL YOU
If you can't remember to drink a glass of water every hour or two, set your cell phone to ring every hour as a reminder.

4. EAT FRUIT EVERY DAY
Fruit can be eighty percent water or more, so if you eat several pieces of fruit a day (as you should), you get an extra glass of water.

5. INSTALL WATER COOLERS
People are more likely to get a drink if there is a water cooler than if there is only a tap.

TAKING ACTION

Choose at least one action you can take to drink more water each day.

ACTION:

KEY 7 MINDFUL EATING

Every time you get a snack for your children, you take a bite for yourself. When you bake a cake, you wouldn't dream of eating a piece, but you lick clean the bowl and the icing knife. You rarely order dessert, but you often ask your husband if you can have a bite of his. Sound familiar?

These are all bad eating habits that I've gotten into in the past through mindlessness. My conscious mind told me that I ate responsibly, and if you looked at my three main meals, I did. But there was a lot of extra eating going on every day that I wasn't even aware of.

I got rid of my bad food habits by making the commitment that every piece of food I put in my mouth would be a conscious decision. That is harder than it sounds. A shocking number of calories we consume every day come independent of hunger. Here's the classic example: When you watch TV at night, you have "a little something" to keep your hands and mouth busy.

Are we all simply moral failures? Weaklings who can't control our gluttony? I don't think so. We live in a unique time. Never before in human history has so much food been available so cheaply all the time.

We must keep our guard up against this constant whisper to eat, eat, eat. As I explained in Key 1, few of us can do it by will-power alone, so we need to call on God to help us be mindful at all times.

What is mindful eating? It's simply being present—really present—whenever you choose to put food or drink in your mouth. It means asking yourself, "Am I hungry? Do I really want this?" One of the most revealing questions to ask is "Does this even taste good?" It can be amazing how often you will say "no" about some food you were about to put in your mouth.

It is also amazing how often we eat when we're not hungry. Most of us are clock-eaters: we have breakfast, lunch, and dinner every day, at pretty much the same time, regardless of hunger.

If you start to be truly present when you eat, and pay attention to how many items you are tempted to put into your mouth just because they are available, you will start detecting all the unconscious impulses your body has in reaction to food, and you'll learn to control them.

Don't Get Discouraged

Like anything else, mindful eating is a skill that takes practice to perfect. The more you do it, the better you will get, but there will be some bumps along the road. No matter how disciplined we are, we all backslide occasionally.

If you keep working at mindful eating, you will get better at it and will backslide less. But you will still slip now and then, so don't beat yourself up when you do.

FIVE WAYS TO BE A MINDFUL EATER

1. HOW YOU FEEL AFTERWARD

How many of your "feeling bad sessions" are connected to bad food you ate earlier that day or the previous evening? Junk food exists only because people don't sense the connection between what they eat and how they feel. Once you get good at being mindful of this, you'll be amazed at how it changes your eating habits.

2. SAY GRACE

Thanking God for the bounty on your table is the best way I know to immediately bring yourself into a more healthy relationship with your food. If you have a tendency to overeat, ask God to help you. Remind yourself that you are eating for two, you and the Holy Spirit, since your body is His temple. Don't shortchange Him!

3. DON'T MULTITASK WITH FOOD

When you eat . . . eat. When you work . . . work. You will enjoy life so much more if you will do one thing at a time and give it your full attention. Many people are so used to having food around that they come to think of it like they do background noise.

4. SLOW DOWN

It takes about twenty minutes for food to pass through your stomach and reach your small intestine, which sends the "full" message to your brain. If you eat too fast, you will overeat before your brain is signaled that your stomach is full.

5. TURN OFF THE "BARGAIN" DETECTOR

Food is plentiful and inexpensive, and there are all kinds of deals–"supersize," "family packs," "all you can eat." But once you eat beyond what you need, the only deal you receive is a cut rate on diabetes or cardiovascular disease.

TAKING ACTION

Choose at least one action you can take to eat more mindfully.

ACTION:

KEY 8 CURB YOUR SPIRITUAL HUNGER

I am sure you don't need me to convince you of the dangers of smoking, or the terrible cost of drug and alcohol addiction. We're all aware that such substances are pleasure shortcuts.

But people are less aware that food can play the same role. When we turn to food for comfort, we establish a pattern that is unhealthy and even dangerous—and still leaves us without the comfort we seek.

Food addiction is easy, because food doesn't come with the same stigmas as cigarettes or drugs. Unlike these vices, food has a legitimate—even essential—role in health. Only when it slips into overuse does it become a problem. But it's so easy to get to that point! Food is reliable. Unlike spouses, friends, or great weather, it is always there. And that's the problem. Any time we feel spiritually empty, whether through sadness, depression, or boredom, it's easy to reach for food to fill that void. Soon we mistake spiritual hunger for physical hunger, and food becomes the immediate answer to any drop in well-being.

Fortunately, there is another source of comfort that is always there when you need it. That something is God. He is called the "Father of sympathy and the God of every comfort, who consoles us in every trouble" (2 Corinthians 1:3,4).

When I hurt, I have learned to turn to God first, instead of another person or substance. Learning this habit will do more to keep your mind and body sound and your life on an even keel than anything I know.

Today's Spiritual Famine

Today more people are spiritually malnourished than ever before. People get caught up with making money to buy bigger homes and spiffier cars, or with following the latest trends. Time for church or religious matters, or even for spending quiet time in nature, is pushed aside by busy schedules and entertainment.

Caught up in this lifestyle, many people mistake the void they feel inside for physical hunger. They were never taught to recognize spiritual hunger, or what to do about it if they do recognize it.

Even those who do know better and make the effort to be good Christians can get swept up in this spiritual famine, because so many entertainment venues are closed to us. Sometimes there are not many parties we can attend and not many movies we can watch without feeling debased. We assume food is one of the few entertainments open to us that is free from sin, only to fall into the trap of gluttony, which God's Word definitely condemns.

Take a good, hard look inside and decide whether your eating comes from spiritual hunger.

Why Bother?

If you have a rich spiritual life, you'll already be satisfied with the moment, the day, the year, and won't feel the need to "supplement" the moment with food.

We all have these moments at times. You wander through a summer field of fireflies and suddenly feel still and awed by the beauty of it all. The moment is complete in itself. You don't think, "My heart is full of joy and boy do I wish I had a slice of chocolate cake in my hand!" We should reach for those transcendent moments more often than we do, and I think we spend too little time trying to achieve them.

FIVE WAYS TO NOURISH YOUR SPIRIT

1. STOP LYING

If you need to, admit to yourself that your spirit is not getting what it needs from life. Try to identify the sources of emptiness that drive you to bad habits. What can you do to start filling those empty areas with activities or people that will help feed your spirit and connect you with God?

2. ASK

God loves you so much and wants to help you, but you need to ask Him to. The next time you are tempted to eat because you're upset or sad, say "no" out loud. Then go sit quietly for a moment and ask God to help you in your situation.

3. CROWD OUT THE BAD HABITS

Fill your life with so many positive, spiritually reaffirming things that there's no room for anything else. Exercise is a terrific way to fill time with healthy activity that leaves your spirit high and your body recharged.

4. SUPPORT PROGRAMS

Breaking the habit of anesthetizing your spiritual hunger with food or other substances is tough. Support groups aren't for everyone, but many who were skeptical at first found success this way.

5. GIVE IT SOME TIME

Don't plan on instant success. Commit fiercely to your success, but love yourself no matter what happens. You will have some slips but you will have more successes.

TAKING ACTION

Choose at least one action you can take to nourish your spirit.

ACTION:

KEY 9 DE-STRESS

There's a dangerous drug out there.

It makes your heart race, constricts your blood vessels, raises your blood pressure, turns off your short-term memory and other nasty things.

I bet you'd go out of your way to steer clear of this drug. Yet you give yourself doses of it every day. I was addicted for years. The drug is cortisol. It is the most famous of the glucocorticoids, the stress drugs your body makes daily.

Stress is the opposite of relaxation. Physically, it is your body gearing up to tackle whatever situation has arisen. And it does by sending stress hormones, like cortisol, in all directions. If you lead a typical modern life, stress hormones are triggered not just every day but every hour.

What Happens to Us Under Stress

In the past, most societies were centered around the slow rhythms of agriculture and the seasons. There was the occasional war or flood, but for the most part, life was low-stress.

Stressful events required a physical response—battling an invader, staying afloat in a flood. In those circumstances, the stress hormones sent to your body are needed. They sharpen your senses, increase your pain threshold, reduce your ability to think rationally, and divert energy from digestion to the cardiovascular system, causing your blood pressure to rise and respiration and heart rate to increase.

In a life-and-death struggle, these physiological changes are crucial, but they come at a cost, particularly when they are triggered on a daily basis. Chronic stress doesn't allow the body to recover, and slowly kills it.

A GUIDE TO STRESS-RELATED DISEASE

Cardiovascular Disease

Here is the overall impact of stress on your cardiovascular system. It gives you thick, syrupy blood that is likely to clot. This pushes through your pounding heart and narrowed blood vessels and therefore causes your heart to work harder. People with heart disease are four times as likely to suffer a heart attack if they are chronically stressed.

Diabetes

Adrenaline (triggered by stress) signals your fat cells to send their fat into your blood stream, where it can be converted into glucose for your muscles. Your body tries to keep as much fat and glucose in your blood as possible during stress. To do this, it overrides your insulin, which is trying to force the fat and glucose into storage or muscle tissue. (The only places it doesn't override the insulin are muscles being used right then, which need all the glucose they can get.) Since insulin-resistance is the main problem for diabetes, stress makes it worse.

Weight Gain

Cortisol from your adrenal glands, triggered by stress, stimulates the appetite. It makes you ravenous, and it makes fat storage extra easy, especially around the abdomen.

Ulcers and Digestive Disorders

Normally, your stomach wall is lined with a thick layer of mucus to protect it from the hydrochloric acid that breaks down food in the stomach. But when your digestion is frequently shut down by stress, your body can get out of step with making mucus to coat the stomach. Then the acid burns a hole in an unprotected spot on the stomach wall, and presto, you've got an ulcer.

Immunity and Aging

If your stress is chronic, cortisol keeps reducing your white blood cells until your immune system is depleted. Suddenly you are more likely to catch colds and other diseases.

Under chronic stress, your body stops repairing its cells, and instead uses its protein as an extra source of fuel for the "fight or flight" situation it is sensing. All body maintenance projects cease. That's why people with long-term stress look run down. They are breaking down on a cellular level.

FIVE WAYS TO DE-STRESS YOURSELF

1. SOCIAL SUPPORT
Social isolation leads to elevated cortisol levels. Hanging around with others is one of the best ways to make us feel good and relaxed.

2. SHRUG THERAPY
How you react to things you can't control helps determine your stress level and quality of health. People who can shrug off the

small things and things they can't control do a lot better. The Bible calls it "casting your care."

3. FIND YOUR ELEMENT—AND STAY THERE

You may be in a position that doesn't make you happy and you need to make a change. You may be happy with your position, but if it steals your health, get out as fast as you can! Your element is waiting for you out there somewhere; if you aren't in it, go find it now!

4. NUTRITION, SUPPLEMENTS, AND DIET

Stress can cause your body to deplete certain vitamins more rapidly than others. If you are under heavy stress, supplements can be helpful.

5. RELAXATION TECHNIQUES

Relaxation is not selfish or slacking off. It is a way of recharging your batteries. The possibilities for relaxation are endless, but here are some favorites: play, laughter, exercise, sleep, prayer, massage, time in the outdoors. What's your favorite?

TAKING ACTION

Choose at least one action you can take to reduce your stress load.

ACTION:

KEY 10 RIGHT VISION

To get somewhere you have to know where you are going. You may not know the exact route, but you at least have a goal in mind.

In your effort to enjoy the healthy life you deserve, you need to have a vision of your goal. What will your life be like when you are eating well, and you feel fit, comfortable, and happy? What will you look like? What kinds of activities will fill your days? Only when you have a vision of the new you can you start making the necessary plans to achieve it.

Before we achieve victory, we have to transition from wishing to taking action. God has only one gear: forward! He has no park and no reverse. He wants you to start progressing toward your goals, but before you can do that you must get a clear image of those goals.

FIVE WAYS TO DEVELOP RIGHT VISION

1. THINK (AND SPEAK) YOUR REALITY INTO EXISTENCE

It may sound like something from a contemporary self-help course, but the idea of "manifesting your reality" is straight out of the Bible: "As a man thinks in his heart, so is he" (Proverbs 23:7).

We usually think our problems are ruining our lives, but usually it is our attitude toward them that does the ruining. We have more to do with how our lives turn out than we like to admit. Learning how to think right is mandatory for good health. Thoughts affect emotions, and they both affect the body. In order for you to be whole, you must maintain a healthy mind.

Another excellent practice is to create a vision of the ideal you. Carry this vision around in your head, and assume the role of the ideal you, as if you were acting in a play. Say and do the things the "ideal you" would do, instead of what the "now you" does.

2. MANAGE YOUR FEELINGS

We all have positive and negative emotions, and they can make us feel wonderful or awful. But feelings are fickle and unreliable. God has given us wisdom, and we should walk in it, not emotions. Negative emotions can raise our stress level and lead to illness and disease.

Part of the epidemic of emotions that I see around me may be dietary. Eating low-quality, high-carb diets is associated with quick drops in blood sugar which causes not only hunger but grumpiness, sadness, confusion, and related feelings.

To manage your emotions and manage your life, you need to call on Heaven's wisdom; but to have the clarity of mind to receive Heaven's wisdom, it helps to have good nutrition.

3. ASSUME THE BEST

We can quickly ruin a day with wrong thinking. Replace suspicion and fear with trust. Trust breeds trust. Trusting others, and especially trusting God, helps keep us healthy. When we trust, we are relaxed and at rest.

4. GET THE SMALL THINGS RIGHT

The small things we do have surprisingly powerful repercussions. Small things set the tone for our days. Going the extra mile for people—whether it's a slightly larger tip, an unexpected compliment or gift, or even holding a door for them—costs you little, and gets you a lot.

There are many other ways to get the small things right: keeping yourself attractive, keeping your house clean, keeping your schedule organized. Do all the small things that a person of sincerity, faith, self-respect, and excellence would do, and you'll discover that you are that person!

5. BE A PART OF SOMETHING BIGGER THAN YOURSELF

You will have much more success in all your endeavors if you can make them about something other than YOU. Nothing can make your vision more "right" than knowing that you are working for God's glory. There is much work to do on earth, and a multitude of ways of carrying it forward. Whether it is helping children, spreading the Good News, or raising a family, nothing is more fulfilling or makes doing the right thing easier than knowing that you are part of the grandest vision of them all!

TAKING ACTION

Choose at least one action you can take to develop your vision.

ACTION:

KEY 11 MAKE IT EASY

If you are a person of passion, like me, you are probably chomping at the bit to launch into your new lifestyle, to embrace all of it as fast as possible.

But let me be the first to say whoa! Go slow. Most human beings want everything fast, but God is not in a hurry. He is in this with you for the long haul. He will deliver you from all your bondages little by little. There is a reason I've asked you to take only one action for each key and not five!

I have found that the secret to success in any long-term project is to make it easy. I am not saying that your new program will always be easy, because it won't. Any time we break old bad habits and make new ones that are good for us, it presents challenges. You will definitely have to resist the temptation to give up and be willing to press on during those times when your progress isn't going as fast as you'd like. I am saying that you can make it as easy on yourself as possible.

FIVE WAYS TO MAKE SUCCESS EASY

1. TAKE SMALL STEPS

In the previous section, I talked about the importance of setting your sights on your dreams and goals, and now I'll remind you how essential it is to break down those goals into doable steps.

Plan your short-term goals so you have something within reach to shoot for. Writing them down will give you a sense of whether you are on track. Don't make light of little victories. Small successes breed large ones.

2. LAUGH AT SETBACKS

No matter how carefully you plan your progress, you will have setbacks. One of the big differences between successful and unsuccessful people is not whether they have setbacks, or even the frequency of their setbacks, but how they respond to them. Successful people are able to laugh off setbacks and get right back on the horse.

3. MAKE IT CONVENIENT

If you are a busy person, you will have to find ways to fit the twelve keys into your schedule. Fortunately, there are ways to make all these things convenient. For example, it's easier than ever to find healthy food and choose a hairstyle and clothing that make you feel good about yourself but aren't high maintenance. Do what is simple and enjoy life more!

4. MAKE IT FUN

Be realistic. You will only keep doing things if you enjoy them. God wants us to enjoy life to the full. Find an exercise you like. Find a church where you feel the Spirit of God is present and moving powerfully. Keep the concept of fun in the back of your mind the whole time you work toward a healthy lifestyle, because you aren't getting healthy to make yourself miserable.

5. REWARD YOURSELF

Don't underestimate the power of silly rewards. Treating yourself after you reach that first short-term goal isn't silly if it keeps you motivated! When you have written down your short and long-term goals, include some appropriate rewards for yourself with it. Rewards and celebrations give structure for your journey and let you reflect on what you've accomplished.

TAKING ACTION

Choose at least one action you can take to make your healthy lifestyle extra easy on you.

ACTION:

KEY 12 TAKE RESPONSIBILITY

One of the biggest problems in society today is that people don't want to take responsibility for their lives. They want quick fixes. Society has trained them to believe that if they have problems, somebody else is responsible.

I don't like this passive mentality. Whatever your life is, you must make the best you can out of it.

I'm not saying you are responsible for the current state of your life. Lots of uncontrollable events occur in our lives. The situation you find yourself in may or may not be your fault. But it is your fault if you take it lying down! You do not have to stay in that bad situation. You get to make a choice.

No matter how you got to where you find yourself today, don't let it be an excuse to stay there. I had many excuses and reasons for my poor health, bad attitude, and unbalanced life. As long as I offered excuses, I never made progress.

The Power of Free Will

God will give you all the tools you need on Earth to reach spiritual completion. When you are in the depths of self-pity, free will can feel awful, a pressure and a responsibility you just don't want. But once you make the commitment to maintain your body and soul as you should, you discover that free will is your most valuable possession.

This is why you must avoid self-pity at all costs. Self-pity is an emotion that feeds on itself and steals your power. You need power to become the person you were meant to be, and you cannot be pitiful and powerful at the same time. I had a major problem with self-pity in my earlier years, and not until I stopped feeling sorry for myself did I start making progress.

We feel better about ourselves when we approach life boldly, ready to be accountable and responsible. Through God you are ready for anything. Confront your life head on and never turn back.

One Way to Take Responsibility for Your Life

Up until now I've given you five action options. When it comes to taking responsibility for your own life, there is no wiggle room. The time has come to be very honest with yourself and with God. You either do it or you don't. Make the decision to do so. When you have a moment of privacy, take a deep breath, clear your head, and repeat this phrase:

"I am responsible for my own life. No one can take charge of it but me. If I am unhappy or unhealthy, I know I have the power to change that. I have all the help and knowledge I need, and with God's hand today I start becoming the person of excellence I have always known I could be."

Congratulations. Thanks for taking this journey with me, and blessings on you for the exciting and wondrous journey you are just beginning.

TAKING ACTION

Choose to take charge of your life. Write down your decision, commit to it, and begin today.

ACTION: